A BETTER WAY SERIES

A NEW PERSPECTIVE

A Journey of Brain Health, Faith, and Well-being

CRAIG BOOKER

Ⓑ BOOKER & CO

A New Perspective
Copyright © 2025 by Craig Booker

Published by Booker & Co, LLC
Edmond, Oklahoma
bookerandco.org

Printed in the United States of America

First edition

Library of Congress Control Number: 2025913974

ISBN: 979-8-9989757-0-7 (ebook)

ISBN: 979-8-9989757-1-4 (international trade paper edition)

All rights reserved. No part of this publication may be reproduced, stored or transmitted in any form or by any means, electronic, mechanical, photocopying, recording, scanning, or otherwise without written permission from the publisher. It is illegal to copy this book, post it to a website, or distribute it by any other means without permission.

The Information such as phone numbers, URLs or internet addresses (websites, blogs, etc.) in this book are offered as a resource. The author and the publisher expressly disclaim responsibility for the persistence or accuracy of URLs or internet addresses (websites, blogs, etc.) referred to in this book. They are not intended in any way to be or imply an endorsement by the author or publisher.

Designations used by companies to distinguish their products are often claimed as trademarks. All brand names and product names used in this book and on its cover are trade names, service marks, trademarks and registered trademarks of their respective owners. The publishers and the book are not associated with any product or vendor mentioned in this book. None of the companies referenced within the book have endorsed the book.

This book is written as a source of information only. The information contained in this book should by no means be considered a substitute for the advice, decisions or judgment of the reader's professional, medical or financial advisors. All efforts have been made to ensure the accuracy of the information contained in this book as of the date published. The author and the publisher expressly disclaim responsibility for any adverse effects arising from the use or application of the information contained herein.

Unless indicated otherwise, scripture quotations are from the Holy Bible, New Living Translation. © 1996, 2004, 2015 by Tyndale House Foundation. Used by permission of Tyndale House Publishers, Inc., Carol Stream, Illinois 60188. All rights reserved.

Scripture quotations labeled NIV are from The Holy Bible, New International Version®, NIV®. Copyright © 1973, 1978, 1984, 2011 by Biblica, Inc.® Used by permission of Zondervan. All rights reserved worldwide. www.Zondervan.com. The "NIV" and "New International Version" are trademarks registered in the United States Patent and Trademark Office by Biblica, Inc.®

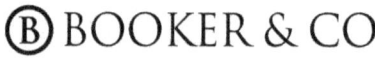

This book is dedicated to my wife, Kristi. The journey has been long, but you never gave up on me. Your dedication to my dreams and well-being exceeds anything I could have imagined when we said, "I do!" Thank you for loving me when I was falling apart. You have supported me through all of my wild ideas and countless career changes. When others might have left, you chose to stay. Thank you for believing in me when I didn't believe in myself. I love you more each day.

Contents

Author's Note vii
Introduction xi

1. Understanding Fear 1
2. What Got Me Here 7
3. Milestones, Waypoints, & Life Lessons 25
4. Wellness, Well-being, & Why They Matter ... 39
5. Conversations for Good 49

Conclusion 81
Acknowledgments 89
Notes 93
About the Author 95

Author's Note

When I first faced serious brain health issues, my wife and I had no idea where to turn. I wrote this book to serve as the resource I wish I had during those initial weeks, months, and years of battling brain health challenges. It's also worth noting that I intentionally kept this book short.

Several years ago, I finished a first draft of this book that was much longer. I soon realized that most of my intended readers aren't avid readers. In other words, most of you usually don't read long books for fun or list reading as a hobby. This isn't a jab at you; it's just a realization I had while writing that made me go back to the drawing board.

I wanted to create a book that the average reader could finish from cover to cover in a few hours and find the resources they needed. Focusing on my audience changed everything about the book, although some content, like stories or explanations of my experiences, remained the same.

Everyone faces challenges with brain health. Yes, you read that right—everyone. For some, these problems are rare and minor, while for others, they may feel overwhelming. Many of you might be somewhere in the middle. No matter where you stand on this spectrum, we all have work to do.

While some may deal with minor annoyances infrequently, others' lives have been disrupted by mental health issues. Still, some lovingly support friends or family members facing various levels of brain health challenges. I wrote this book to provide you with what I didn't have many years ago. Understand that, like me, this book is an imperfect work in progress.

AUTHOR'S NOTE

My prayer for you is that by the end of this book, you will have a new perspective on mental health, also called brain health. I use the term brain health because it provides a clearer picture of what many people experience. Using the term mental health isn't wrong; I just prefer how brain health makes me think differently.

After finishing my first draft, I realized that the resources I had to share were better suited for a series of short books. This book is the first in the A Better Way series. If you find this book helpful, please visit craigbooker.com to learn more about upcoming releases in the series.

If you're dealing with brain health issues, remember you're not meant to face them alone. To connect with people who understand what you're going through, visit overflow.community. Joining the community is free. I created Overflow to be the community I wish I had years ago. I hope you'll check it out.

Introduction

Helpless & Hopeless

I remember the first time I realized that things would never be the same again. Despite having a wonderful and loving wife, friends, and family, I felt all alone. I realized I had never known anyone who struggled to cope with everyday life at this level. My newfound circumstances led me to ask, "What was wrong with me?" and "Who do I call for help?"

For two years, I scrambled to find a stable job. After being laid off in 2002, I became intimately familiar with my vulnerability. As a newlywed, I did everything possible to provide my beautiful bride with a loving and stable life. However, my efforts to find work felt inadequate, and I struggled to cope with the challenges of my early adulthood.

I felt **helpless** because I could not take action. I was utterly overwhelmed by my new reality and the daunting task of finding the right person to call. I was battling this new reality so much that I would never measure up. I'm not saying I was a victim or that I had it any worse than the next person. I just had no clue what the first step toward recovery might be.

INTRODUCTION

I felt **hopeless** because I believed I had failed my wife, family, and God. As a newly married man, I had been holding on for dear life, white-knuckling my way through life. I felt like I had turned in my man card the moment I couldn't keep it all together anymore. It was all too much, and nothing, not even my deeply rooted faith, could keep me afloat. I found my head slipping below the water's surface with no one in sight to lend a hand.

Plotting The Course

If you are anything like I was, you may feel overwhelmed by the weight of your struggle. Where do you start when you cannot keep your head above water? What does it look like to recover from trauma and brokenness? Should I call a doctor, a pastor, a psychologist, a psychiatrist, or a counselor?

You might worry about what this means for you or your family. Is this what they mean when they say someone has lost it? Am I going crazy? What will people think of me when they learn that I had a sudden breakdown? I found myself with more questions than answers. If you are anything like me, you might be looking for a roadmap or, even better, a modern-day GPS app to guide you. We need to slow down and take a moment to pause. Before moving forward, and long before seeing a doctor or counselor, most people need a change in perspective. The path for someone healing from mental health, also known as brain health challenges, is unlike any other. It's a long journey with a lot of work to do.

INTRODUCTION

What I learned the hard way is that you will be devastated if you approach this as you might on a road trip or when planning a summer vacation. First, each person is unique, and there are no direct flights. The healing and recovery process does not follow a linear path from point A to point B.

> You might ask, "Who said anything about recovery? I just want to return to life like it used to be." Hold that thought.

Before diving into the book, let's chart our course. This one is personal. After all, there is a good reason you chose to spend your time reading or listening to this instead of doing something else. So, how can you maximize your investment? How will this book help you or someone you love struggling with fear?

Let's begin by clarifying what this book is not. This book is not a magic pill. I will not present three easy steps to heal from fear, anxiety, depression, or other brain health challenges. This journey is unique for each individual and should not be oversimplified. I will share aspects of my journey with you and the lessons God has taught me.

God does instantly heal people from their anxiety or depression in some cases. Up to this point in my life, this has not been my experience. I have repeatedly prayed for God to take it away, but I continue to live with it daily. Rather than obsessing over why God has not healed me, I have focused on my path toward healing and recovery.

INTRODUCTION

Who Should Read This?

When I think of this book, I generally picture two groups of individuals: those who struggle with fear, anxiety, and depression, and those standing beside them. I envision a friend or family member learning to care for someone overwhelmed by brain health challenges. These personas may seem cliché, but they help guide my efforts and inform me about the resources to include in this book.

For those individuals facing brain health challenges, I hope this book provides you with the encouragement, inspiration, community, and resources essential for your journey. You have likely faced trauma and challenges far beyond what many can imagine. Whether you have just discovered anxiety or have been on this path for years, this book is meant for you.

For all the friends and family members who chose this book to help you better understand what a friend or family member is experiencing, I applaud you. Genuinely striving to understand is one of the most generous things you can do for someone close to you.

To Be Understood

Those who struggle with anxiety often feel lonely and profoundly misunderstood. They do not wish to be fixed like one might repair a broken car. Instead, they seek to be understood and accepted just as they are. Regardless of the outcome, they want to know you love them beyond their diagnosis. To be seen and, more importantly, understood is to love the individual. They want to be loved in the middle of their mess, just as Jesus famously did for many.

INTRODUCTION

How do I know all of this? These were my thoughts and desires while I was deeply entrenched in a battle with anxiety and depression.

More Than Just A Book

I am here to advocate for brain health. This book is my way of bringing the discussion of fear and anxiety into the mainstream. It serves as an act of generosity and a means of helping others. I have carefully structured the material to help you maximize your investment. My goal is to update the content as I learn, create a vibrant community, and build a continuous supply of resources.

Why Write This Book?

As a student of brain health, I regularly seek new perspectives on anxiety and depression. Most of the content I encounter includes part of a person's story, or what many might call a memoir. Inevitably, it details how they miraculously overcame their battles with fear, anxiety, or depression. When I come across one, I am instantly enthralled and eager to consume everything the author has written. I hope to read something new that I have never encountered before.

While the author's account often inspires me, I also feel a sense of longing. Please don't misunderstand me; there is always value in someone's story of fear, anxiety, and depression. Hearing about a person's trials and the victories they achieve is incredibly important. These podcasts, articles, and books inspire others and help reduce mental health stigma. All of this is beneficial.

INTRODUCTION

I rarely encounter personal accounts of individuals who continue to live with fear, anxiety, or depression. I am what many call a hopeless romantic or an eternal optimist. I appreciate a good happily-ever-after story as much as the next person, but brain health doesn't always work that way. More often than not, fear, anxiety, and depression persist. Their lives remain messy, and they continue to struggle. We need to hear more of these stories.

Let's face it. People, myself included, seek quick and easy solutions to their struggles. We want answers when we purchase a book! Why are search results flooded with articles listing three easy steps to overcome addiction or five principles to live by while fighting fear? The simple truth is that these headlines motivate people to read an article or buy a book.

What happens to someone who prays endlessly to remove anxiety, and God says either, "No," or "Not yet?" How does this person face another day? How do they continue to have faith when God doesn't take away the hurt and suffering?

These questions are for the rest of us—those still waiting on God's healing, those who do not have it all together, and those who feel fear yet faithfully continue their struggle. They are for people who face overwhelming anxiety or crippling depression and choose to place their faith in God. This book is for those who experience doubts about their faith, God's plan, and sometimes His goodness.

INTRODUCTION

My Prayer For You

My friend, I pray for God's miraculous healing over you or your friend's life. I pray that fear, dread, and anxiety will cease. I ask God to provide you comfort that lasts longer than a moment. I long to hear about God's power rewiring your brain. I want to see you encouraging those who are still battling, reminding them that their day of healing is coming.

Until that day, I want you to know that you are never alone. First, the Bible tells us that God is always with us (Isaiah 41:10, Psalms 16:8). I walk alongside you, praying for a miracle for both of us. You are not alone in your struggle. I ask God to grant me wisdom, tools, and tips to encourage you along this path. I am grateful for the bond we share because of our struggle.

> "So do not fear, for I am with you; do not be dismayed, for I am your God. I will strengthen you and help you; I will uphold you with my righteous right hand."
> Isaiah 41:10 NIV

> "I know the Lord is always with me. I will not be shaken, for he is right beside me."
> Psalms 16:8 NLT

INTRODUCTION

A Better Way

The phrase "A Better Way" transcends being a cheesy cliché used to describe a superior solution. It serves as a statement of faith, choosing to believe in God's goodness and the abundant life that the Bible promises us while rejecting the narrative of "You will always be this way." In the context of this book and mental health, it involves actively deciding what we believe, how we perceive our world, and how we lead our lives.

As I stated, A Better Way involves actively deciding what we believe, how we perceive our world, and how we lead our lives. It does not imply naively viewing the world through rose-colored glasses. Instead, it signifies believing in God's goodness and His unique plan for our lives. Similarly, it is not a precise formula, a three-step plan, or ten quick tips to heal from mental health challenges. While this is merely the introduction, I hope you will join me in pursuing A Better Way.

1

Understanding Fear

As I awaken to a pitch-black room, I find myself lost, wondering why I am awake and where I am. Fear races through my body, as if trying to intimidate the blood coursing through my veins. I am cold and shivering, and it is still dark outside. Everything in me tells me to get back into the safety of my bed, and I feel lost as to the time of day. I glance at my phone and quickly realize it's early morning, and I already feel so behind. I cannot escape the fear that I awoke to what seems like only moments ago.

My brain is on high alert, keenly focused on my protection—the lens of fear coloring my vision. I hear creaks and pops and wonder if an intruder is in my home. I pause for a moment to question whether I am in danger. I quickly realize it is just the house settling. I look outside my window into the darkness and see objects lurking in the shadows. I look again, only to discover that whatever I saw was merely a figment of my imagination.

A NEW PERSPECTIVE

As I head to the bathroom, listening for signs of impending doom, I realize I am in no real danger. I wonder what has triggered my body's defenses, but I reassure myself that I will be alright if I make it to the bathroom. Closing the door, I relax, and the fear overwhelming my mind slips away. I must have had an intense dream, and this Spirit of Fear is only temporary.

As evening approaches, I'm reminded of the terror I felt less than twenty-four hours ago. The fear that consumed my thoughts still lingers. I'm intrigued by how my mind transitioned so rapidly from constant vigilance, anticipating disaster, to relaxation and calm. What enabled this shift? Is it possible for me to replicate the process? Can I help my brain escape fight-or-flight mode? I find myself with more questions than answers.

Why Tell This Story?

Fear and anxiety affect humans on many different levels. While many can relate to having a bad dream, most do not live with a spirit of fear constantly hanging over their heads. This true story illustrates how quickly fear can take hold of our thoughts and feelings. It distinctly portrays how fear appears and slips away without us realizing why or how.

Our bodies are equipped with a built-in alert system known as the amygdala. When our brain detects danger, it floods the body with a stress hormone called cortisol. This process helps us respond quickly to steer clear of dangerous situations. This system is beneficial; it keeps us alive.

All people undergo this process when their bodies sense danger. Once the threat subsides, our bodies turn off the alarm and return to a normal state. We go about our day prepared to react if danger arises again. This is how God designed us.

So, what would you do if your body never slowed down from this fight-or-flight response? Your body continues to secrete cortisol, and your brain persistently searches for the next big disaster. Life-altering trauma may be just around the corner, or is it? I know what it's like to live in a healthy relationship with fear, and I have experienced how it feels to view everything through the lens of fear. While I don't have all the answers, I will share what I wish I had known earlier.

Expectations For This Book

In the chapters ahead, I will explore what it is like to live with anxiety from the perspective of an imperfect follower of Jesus Christ. While I hope this is helpful to all readers, those who do not believe in Jesus Christ might find my explanations frustrating or simply intolerable. Still, I hope readers can find comfort in hearing my story, the wisdom I have gained, and what God has revealed to me through my journey.

I have tried many forms of treatment, and while many have helped, they fall short on their own. Jesus has shown us a better way to live, which offers us peace, healing, and an abundant life. Craig Groeschel suggests that we can discover the life we long for by examining how Jesus lived. Just as Jesus teaches us ways to refocus our attention on what matters, his life also models a healthy relationship with fear.

Living A Life Of Fear

I've been there. I have lived every moment anticipating the worst, waiting for various forms of loss, scarcity, or regret. I know what it is like to be overwhelmed by trauma, to the extent that every situation seems negative. One traumatic event after another, until you wonder if your world will ever stop spinning.

A NEW PERSPECTIVE

And then, abruptly, it **STOPS**.

Like hitting a wall, the disastrous momentum comes to a stop. For a brief moment, you question whether it will start up again. Once the dust clears, you cautiously emerge from your shell to look for any signs of danger. Finding none, you drift off into a deep sleep, weary from the descent.

As you awaken from slumber, you look around with skeptical wonder. Seeing no signs of doom, you begin to step out from the safety of your bed. Seeking solutions, you consult trusted professionals for wisdom, a roadmap, or a set of next steps. You wonder if this is forever or merely a season of your life you will look back on.

My Prayer

Here is my prayer for you. If you or someone you love is at this point, I pray God surrounds you with friends and a team of professionals who firmly believe that recovery is possible. Someone who never gives up hope, believing God has a fulfilling life ahead of you. No matter how bleak the situation appears, I pray this group is there to cheer you on and encourage you to believe in God's best for your special someone.

Application Questions

1. In the chapter, I describe waking up in fear and gradually realizing there was no real danger. Have you ever experienced something similar? How did you calm yourself down in that situation?

2. The text mentions that our bodies have a built-in alarm system, known as the amygdala, which triggers the release of cortisol throughout the body when danger is detected. How might understanding this biological process help someone dealing with frequent anxiety or fear?

3. In the chapter, I said, "Jesus has shown us a better way to live, which offers us peace, healing, and abundant life." What are your thoughts on this perspective? Do you think spirituality or faith can play a role in managing anxiety and fear?

4. The chapter ends with a prayer for those struggling with fear and anxiety. What support systems or resources do you think are most beneficial for individuals facing these challenges? How important is it to have people who "never give up hope" when someone is going through difficult times?

2

What Got Me Here

Reflecting on my past, I gently remind myself that it hasn't always been this way. I remember a time in my life when my thoughts felt like a much safer place to visit—a space where things weren't overshadowed by what might happen. It was a time when my first instinct wasn't to think of the worst-case scenario. The world and my thoughts felt like a safer place back then.

Chronic fear and anxiety surfaced in my late twenties. Before that, I believe I had a healthy relationship with fear. I was familiar with these emotions, but they never lingered for long. I might experience anxiety before a big test or meeting, which I consider typical.

Until my late twenties, mental illness was something that happened to others, not to me. I hope to share the details that have led me to where I am today.

A NEW PERSPECTIVE

Other events, circumstances, and trauma contribute to my story, but I will begin here for simplicity.

It was 2001, and I was newly married, working full-time as a web developer for a local startup. The term "web developer" did not exist then, and everything I worked on seemed to be breaking new ground. A few years prior to starting full-time, I worked for a small local company with a maximum of ten employees. I started part-time but eagerly jumped on the opportunity to go full-time when a position became available. This job was what I affectionately referred to as my first "real job."

In my mind, I was getting paid a good amount of money to play—I mean, work on a computer. My work was new and exciting, and I was working alongside some of the brightest, most gifted people I've ever met. It was early 2001, and the financial markets were struggling. As a small startup, we succeeded in going public. However, the company needed additional funding to grow. In retrospect, our financial situation was worse than it appeared.

It was only a short time before the executive team announced that a company from Sunnyvale, California, had acquired our startup. Here I was, figuring out my identity and grappling with the usual challenges of startup life. A new opportunity emerged to train and certify two other groups of developers to create our core product. The opportunity seemed exciting, so I accepted the role and joined the training department in California. Little did I know that this transition would eventually leave me vulnerable.

Shortly after 9/11, the financial markets were tough, and we were acquired by one of our largest customers. It was strange, and the process was more involved than I let on, so I will save you the details. I had about a year left to complete my bachelor's degree in Business Management. I was working full-time, and my wife, Kristi, was about to start full-time as a nurse after finishing school. I took the semester off to adjust to working full-time. All in all, things were going well.

It was around this time that things at work began to take an unusual turn. I was now part of the training department. My former managers were no longer my bosses, and we were now a part of a large company. Our fearless CEO was now managing what had once been his company.

Corporate America was unsettling for our former CEO. He did not fit into the bureaucracy of corporate life. His team still had jobs, but his hands were essentially tied. I deeply admire and respect him for doing what was best for the team, but it crushed me to see him in this state.

One day, I received an email from one of my former managers who worked at the Oklahoma City office. My former manager warned me of things he had heard. The company was in poor financial shape and was laying off workers deemed nonessential to the business. Since I was part of the training team, I was now considered an expendable employee. The day was an absolute blur, but by its end, I found myself without a job.

My New Vulnerability

Post-9/11, the job market was in the worst shape I had ever seen. I was unemployed and struggling to find work. I'll save you the unemployment stories for now, but I felt completely lost. Jobs as a web developer were almost nonexistent in Oklahoma City, leaving me uncertain about the future of my career.

A NEW PERSPECTIVE

Here I was, trying to figure out how to provide for my family. I was still somewhat new to the idea of a two-income household. Kristi, my wife, had been employed full-time for a short time. It was brief enough that it hardly registered in my memory. I was told I would receive unemployment benefits, but how long would that last?

After reviewing my options with Kristi, we decided that I should work towards completing my bachelor's degree while also looking for a job. Schoolwork would occupy my time as I applied for various positions. I would call the unemployment office weekly to report on what felt like an endless job search. Eventually, the unemployment office believed I could use some help, so I had to attend an all-day seminar at the local unemployment office.

My job search left me feeling depressed and hopeless about my future. Although my education was progressing, it seemed to drag on. As part of my coursework, I began an internship that led me to work at an employment agency. While there, I learned that my business degree was too general to lead me anywhere on its own. It certainly would not secure me a job, which left me with a sense of hopelessness.

My internship was coming to an end, and graduation was just a few months away. I was still unemployed and feeling hopeless when my internship ended. I received a call from the employment agency about an opportunity in the Human Resources department at a local call center. The role would involve screening call center employees for a national cellular provider. Excited about any work, I accepted it!

Outsourced

The call center was one of the most sterile corporate environments I had ever experienced. I was nearing the completion of a year-long job assignment and eagerly awaiting a permanent offer from the call center. I had formed several great friendships and was beginning to feel like part of the team when I received the news: they would not be making me an offer or renewing my contract. They were outsourcing the role to another employment agency.

Shortly after being let go, the employment agency contacted me, requesting that I return to their office. They reasoned that if they could get to know me better, they could find me a job. After the usual employment testing, they informed me that they had no opportunities fitting my skill set. Instead, they offered me a temporary position in their office.

I worked at the agency's office recruiting for another cellular call center. My colleagues and I consistently exceeded our goals. I excelled at sourcing candidates, but my boss repeatedly misled me about the potential for permanent employment. Numerous empty promises led me to submit my notice. It was time to move on.

It felt good to stand up for myself. I was extremely frustrated with my job search. I was not interested in holding on, and I had little hope of finding permanent employment. With my wife's support, I left in search of something better. Giving my notice without any opportunities in mind took a huge leap of faith, but I took it.

A New Opportunity

I received a few calls from the employment agency about possible job opportunities over the next several months, one of which sounded promising. I went for an interview, and they offered me the position. I would be interviewing candidates for the warehouse and performing other Human Resource tasks. All in all, I felt hopeful.

My new role in Human Resources appeared to be a good fit. My boss was incredibly kind, and the people were friendly. Finally, I found stable work! Everything was great, except for the actual work.

It soon became clear that the job described in my interview differed from what the employment agency had told me. I was devastated! The role involved minimal recruiting and extensive, repetitive data entry. Over and over, I thought to myself, "What do I do?"

I have to keep this job! It was not a good fit, but what else could I do? Over time, I found it increasingly challenging to go to work. I caught myself staring off into space more often. My boss noticed this and asked if I was alright. I was desperately trying to escape.

All the signs were right there. I should have paid more attention. I kept trying to power through. I didn't want to share my struggle with my wife. She was so happy that I had finally found a job! Things were stable, and the last thing I wanted to do was ruin her happiness. I thought I could make this job work.

The Countdown Begins

I found myself counting the minutes. In the morning, I would count down the time until I could leave for lunch. After lunch, I would count the hours until it was time to go home. When I couldn't go out to lunch with others, I stayed at the office and tried to find a way to escape.

It became increasingly challenging to go to work. I would sit outside the office in my car each morning, praying for a miracle. One morning, my phone rang, and when I answered, I heard my boss on the other end of the line.

I could hear the care in her voice as she began asking questions. She was incredibly concerned as she observed my struggle to enter the office. The parking lot was clearly visible from her office window. Unbeknownst to me, my boss had watched as I parked and sat in my car until it was time to go inside. Saying I was struggling would be an understatement.

One day, when it happened, I was supposed to go to lunch with my mom. My lunch plans fell through, and I found myself desperately in need of my usual escape. I went to a nearby fast-food restaurant across the street to try to get away. Instead of distracting myself from my situation, I found it incredibly hard to eat my sandwich.

I found myself unable to eat. I remember reaching out to someone for help, but I don't recall who it was. I took my time returning to the office and went directly into a private office to work, closing the door behind me.

At this point in my life, I had little history of fear or anxiety. Aside from my search for work after being laid off in 2001, my experience with fear was what I would consider normal. I have no recollection of fear affecting my daily activities.

A NEW PERSPECTIVE

I returned to a quiet corner of the office near my desk. It was the afternoon, and I was trying to power through the rest of the day. I reassured myself that if I could make it to the end of the day, everything would be fine.

A strange feeling washed over me as I began to gain some momentum. I started to ask myself more questions. Could I push my way through? Could I move forward?

A distant thought began to creep ever closer to me. I do not remember calling out to God, but I know He was there. It's interesting how you are aware of someone's presence, yet you can't recall how or when they arrived. I know God was there, but I was too deep inside my head to recognize Him.

A part of me was basking in the hopelessness of my recent job search. I finally found an excellent company to work for, with kind people and a reasonable pay rate. I was so close. Why couldn't I just tolerate the work? Looking back, I wonder if I could have negotiated different job terms. I did not want to give up on it all, but the thought of going to work was eating away at my soul.

I had desperately longed for someone to say "yes." I needed someone to recognize my value and offer me a job. Countless times, I recall feeling discouraged by job advertisements that initially seemed so promising. I would prepare my application and resume, submit it, and never hear a word from the company.

I would contact the company, only to find that they would not answer questions about posted positions. How strange! Certainly, someone knew something, but I needed help finding the answers to my questions. The job posting would soon disappear.

What Got Me Here

I remembered going from office to office, job to potential job. I applied for positions and attended interviews, but heard nothing in return. It felt as though the people who posted these jobs did not exist. It was a very bizarre dynamic.

This feeling, initially blurry, gradually became clearer. Strangely, I do not remember contemplating it at lunch, but I had felt it before. Each time I tried to push it away, the thought returned to me.

I COULD NOT DO THIS ANYMORE!

I couldn't, but I had to. I had to keep it together! This overwhelming sense of obligation weighed on me like never before. Part of me said, "Hold on, you got this." Part of me said, "WAIT?!? Are you kidding me?" And then, somewhere in between, something happened!

From this point on, all I remember is talking to my boss. The details of how I managed to get to her office are unclear. I remember breaking down in her office. I lost it. All of my composure was <u>GONE</u>. I knew I could no longer fake it. There would be no more powering through. No self-imposed pep talks to BE STRONG.

I don't know how much time passed, but that didn't matter. My manager called my wife and did her best to explain what had happened. I remember being present, but I felt completely awkward. My manager was incredibly kind and focused on my well-being. Surprisingly, I don't recall any discussion about what we would do regarding work.

A NEW PERSPECTIVE

Enlisting Professional Help

I remember being in a doctor's office, explaining what happened and how I felt. The doctor struggled to speak or understand English, which should have been a sign. At this point, I was too far off the tracks to question others. I just needed help!

I went home and returned to the doctor many times. Each time, it became clear that the doctor did not understand my struggle. With each appointment, I experienced a new set of side effects. It was not getting any better.

I am curious to know how much time has passed. My wife, Kristi, contacted my boss, who recommended a specific outpatient clinic. I went there to fill out paperwork and see what it was like. Things were not improving, and I was desperate for something to work. At that point, I didn't feel safe driving, so my mom drove me instead.

I remember participating in a group therapy session where we shared aspects of our lives. Everyone seemed to have different conditions, which felt overwhelming. Listening to the problems of others only seemed to heighten my anxiety.

My Fear Grows

The fear was eating me alive! I remember pounding. My heart was pounding, and fear clouded my ability to reason. At some point, I began doing all sorts of strange things to cope. I started making odd sounds with my mouth. I had developed a new set of habits — habits I wasn't fond of, but couldn't stop doing.

I distinctly remember being unable to calm down when I left the day clinic. My world was spiraling out of control, and there was little anyone—doctor or otherwise—could do about it.

I remember countless trips to a psychologist that proved to be unfruitful and extremely expensive. I found it eerie how little the Christian psychologist spoke about God during these conversations. I felt more like a case to study than someone he wanted to help.

Reflecting on my sessions with the psychologist, I wonder about the God we discussed. We talked about God, but it was not the God I knew. There was never any mention of reaching out to God for help. I was never encouraged to pray or read the Bible, even though the psychologist knew I was a Christian.

A New Hope

I remember waking up each morning, hoping and praying that this was all a bad dream. I would violently rock back and forth in my bed, unable to stop this rocking sensation. I felt it on the inside and out. It would NOT STOP!

I went outside to take a walk, which only heightened my anxiety. Nothing helped stop the rocking. I tried breathing exercises, but they only seemed to frustrate me with minimal results. My fear had taken over even the deepest parts of my psyche.

I had lost hope that the doctor would be able to help me. Each day, I would crawl out of bed only to watch my wife leave for the day. Separation anxiety would overwhelm my mind as she prepared for work. My obsessive-compulsive disorder (OCD) was at an all-time high, leading me to check everything imaginable.

A NEW PERSPECTIVE

The new habits I had mentioned began to take hold, and we were ready to seek further assistance.

Someone suggested I see another doctor about my medications. I distinctly remember traveling across town with Kristi to visit this new doctor. During the first appointment with the doctor, my symptoms seemed to frighten her. Was I really in such bad shape? Were my coping habits to blame?

I was quite robotic in many ways. My body felt stiff and rigid, which concerned the doctor. These behaviors were known side effects of the medication I was taking. After sharing my story, the doctor provided us with an update on my current condition.

Our first course of action was to discontinue the medications prescribed by my previous doctor. Hopefully, as I weaned off the meds, my robotic-like symptoms would diminish. It would be a process, but eventually, I could start on different medications. These new medications were the "Gold Standard" when treating OCD, anxiety, and depression.

The Gold Standard

I recall hearing this phrase and wondering why the previous doctor was not aware of the "Gold Standard." Did he miss that day of medical school? The new doctor instilled a sense of hope, which was something that both Kristi and I desperately needed. Praise God!

Let us return to the time when I was restlessly rocking in my bed. There was an ever-present need to rock back and forth, back and forth. I needed to rock as much as I needed oxygen. When nothing seemed to stop the rocking, I started to pray. It began with the little things, "God help me sleep." The only time I wasn't anxious was when I was sleeping. This made me want to sleep all the time. Not being able to be in a state of rest is torture.

My fear reached an all-time high. I found it challenging to go outside, and even stepping into the front yard felt overwhelming, making mowing the lawn difficult. My doctor suggested that I try taking a walk around the block during one of our sessions, so this became a new goal of mine.

There were many visits back and forth to the doctor, but for the first time, the weird side effects decreased. Slowly, the rigid movements to which I had become accustomed started to subside. Finally!...something seemed to go right. I was not out of the woods yet, but even the slightest glimmer of hope was just the miracle we needed.

Getting Back On My Feet

So, praying helped ease my rocking. Praise God! But now, what should I do? How can I get back on my feet? What will it look like when I arrive? Up to this point, it had taken all of my energy to get through the day. I wasn't used to thinking about anything else. The highlight of my week was attending church each Saturday.

My wife, Kristi, and my mom continued to care for me, ensuring I took my medications and doing their best to understand. I was making my way out of the house, taking walks around the block, but what else should I do at this point? What hope did I have of leading a "normal" life? Do people recover from obsessive-compulsive disorder (OCD) and anxiety? I had many questions, and different people had different answers.

A NEW PERSPECTIVE

Some people would not answer my questions, regardless of how subtle they were. Some quickly told me that I needed to accept my condition and adjust accordingly. I tried my best to understand what this meant for me. I explored real estate, believing I could set my schedule and make a decent living.

It was something I thought I would enjoy, and I did; however, 2007-2008 was not the ideal time to start a career as a realtor. It was one of the worst financial markets of our time. After one year as a realtor, I broke even financially and decided to look elsewhere for a career, but where?

I was browsing job postings, hoping to find something, when I came across an advertisement for work at Apple retail stores. On a whim, I applied and soon forgot about it. Later in the year, I received a call from Apple regarding the position I had applied for months earlier. Eager for any opportunity, I went through four interviews before landing a job with Apple. I was new to Apple products, having owned only a MacBook Pro for six months before joining the team.

My training was delayed several times. I would get excited, but then I wondered if it would ever happen. My training class finally started around the beginning of the new year. We began training in the mall's basement, which I never knew existed. The trainers were surprisingly enthusiastic about Apple culture and what it meant to work for Apple retail. I spent a couple of weeks in training, which did not involve being in the retail store. What type of retail job was this?! I was no stranger to working in retail. What company in its right mind invests this much in its employees?

My time at Apple was more than just a job; it allowed me to forget about the very idea of employment. I had the unique privilege of helping people every day.

What Got Me Here

It was a job in that I was required to show up when scheduled and got paid, which checked off another box. I also received a lunch break each day, which I would spend escaping the store's busyness.

The escape at Apple was different, though. It was merely a break, a time to rest, eat, and so on. It was not time spent avoiding the work I was doing or needed to do. I valued my breaks, but my job was not detestable either. For once, I enjoyed my work.

In my time working at Apple, I do not recall having issues with my anxiety. I remember hustling to get to work, eager to leave at the end of the day, but it was nothing I couldn't handle. I believe this was a time when God smiled at me. It was not perfect by any means. I had frustrations with my job and other people, but for a brief period, I didn't need to look for or think about finding work. The pay could have been better, but it was not the lowest I've ever had in my lifetime, either. My benefits were rock solid.

I loved my time at Apple. I knew it would not last forever, but for once, my feet felt like they were on solid ground.

A NEW PERSPECTIVE

Application Questions

1. In the chapter, I describe a series of job changes and challenges that contributed to my anxiety. How can career instability or dissatisfaction impact brain health, and what strategies might help someone cope with these pressures?

2. The chapter details my experience with different treatments, including medication and therapy. How important is it to find the right healthcare providers when dealing with mental health issues? What can someone do if they feel their current treatment isn't working?

3. I mention finding relief in prayer and eventually in a job I enjoyed at Apple. How can spiritual disciplines and finding meaningful work contribute to managing anxiety and fear? Can you share any personal experiences with this?

4. Throughout the chapter, I describe the support I received from my wife and family. How crucial is a support system when dealing with brain health challenges? What are some ways people can effectively support loved ones struggling with anxiety or similar issues?

3

Milestones, Waypoints, & Life Lessons

Certain moments stand out as I reflect on various aspects of my life. They highlight the lessons I learned during different seasons. As I reflect on my life, I view these moments as milestones on my journey. They help me gauge how far I've come and inspire me to dream about what God has in store for me.

These moments teach me about life and reveal all that God is doing or has done in my life. One of the many reasons I write is to help me organize my thoughts. Writing and reflecting on these lessons is my way of improving and growing. I hope that by sharing, I can help others understand what God taught me about life, love, and brokenness.

A NEW PERSPECTIVE

If anything, these years of living with anxiety have revealed two significant areas that contribute to my anxiety and depression. Certainly, there are others, but I believe these are particularly important. It was in 2005 when I first began to understand the implications of trauma and how it affects my life. I couldn't have explained it then, but I started recognizing its impact on my body.

Major Contributors To Anxiety
- Trauma
- The way I go about life

Defining and Identifying Trauma

While I can certainly speak about my experience with trauma, I believe it is more helpful to begin with a broader definition.

trauma[1]

1. Serious injury to the body, as from physical violence or an accident.
2. Severe emotional or mental distress caused by an experience.
3. An experience that causes severe anxiety or emotional distress, such as rape or combat.
4. An event or situation that causes great disruption or suffering.

In my journey, identifying trauma is one of the most significant steps toward living a healthier life. Understanding my fear and anxiety began with recognizing past traumatic events. These events serve as waypoints and shape my worldview and influence my decisions each day. Taking the time to identify and process these events enables me to live with greater awareness.

Simply understanding how past events, circumstances, or relationships negatively impact my view of the world better prepares me for the road ahead. This awareness enables me to identify potential obstacles ahead and proactively take steps to navigate the challenging terrain. I cannot always avoid the rough road, but understanding my trauma allows me to invite others into this journey. Knowing I do not face these challenges alone gives me the courage to move forward.

I intimately understand that identifying and processing trauma requires a significant amount of challenging conversations. There is so much potential on the other side of this process, but you have to do the work. I encourage you to invest the time and lean into the struggle. This process worked best for me while under the care and guidance of a counselor. Alternatively, a pastor from your local church may be able to provide similar support during this process.

Properly addressing trauma is not a quick and easy process. What I have mentioned thus far provides a high-level view, and I do not mean to oversimplify the process. I have invested years in identifying and processing the trauma in my life. For this book, I have summarized a portion of my experiences. In a later chapter, I will explore another aspect; however, please be aware that there is much more to this process.

A NEW PERSPECTIVE

Way Of Life

How I choose to live significantly impacts whether anxiety controls my life. Let me emphasize that again: how I choose to live significantly impacts whether anxiety controls my life.

Key Points of Failure

- Living On Your Own
- Not Listening To Your Body
- Ignoring How Habits Impact Mental Health

On Your Own

I often lose sight of the opportunities available to me and others who call the U.S. home. Noble values such as independence and hard work have long been fundamental to Western culture and the American Dream. Television shows like ABC's Shark Tank remind me of these incredible opportunities. The show frequently features stories of immigrants who have struggled to reach the United States in pursuit of the American Dream. These stories serve as a reminder of how blessed I am to call the United States my home.

With all the opportunities available to Americans, I often take values such as independence and hard work too far. As strange as it may sound, too much of a good thing can become harmful. Proverbs 25:16 NLT says, "Do you like honey? Don't eat too much, or it will make you sick." I laugh at this idea because it reminds me of the beloved character Winnie-the-Pooh, yet I often do the same thing.

While it may not be honey, I can't count the number of times I've overdone it at holiday meals. So, why should I be surprised that I do the same thing when I work harder? As believers, God calls us to live a life dependent on Him. Yet, I must continually remind myself that God created me to live in a relationship with Him.

When we pursue God's calling for our lives, relying too heavily on hard work and independence can often lead us down the wrong path. In my experience, this wrong path frequently involves living according to the flesh or depending on human power instead of seeking the Holy Spirit. When things don't go as I expect, it's almost second nature for me to work harder rather than take a moment to pray. Additionally, I often tackle tasks on my own. In most cases, the last thing I remember is that I cannot fulfill my God-given calling alone.

Paul's Direction For Timothy

The Bible contains many examples of ordinary, broken people experiencing fear while following God. In 2 Timothy 1, we see a great example of Paul encouraging Timothy not to let fear hinder his calling. In verse 7 of this passage, Paul clearly instructs Timothy that a Spirit of Fear is not from God. Later, in verse 14, Paul reminds Timothy how believers need the Holy Spirit to live out God's calling for their lives.

Life Lessons From Paul and Timothy

- Fear can be a significant barrier in pursuing our calling.
- A Spirit of Fear is not from God.
- We need the Holy Spirit to fulfill God's calling for our lives.

A NEW PERSPECTIVE

Like Timothy, we were not created to pursue God's calling alone. As followers of Jesus Christ, we are meant not only to depend on what the Holy Spirit brings, such as power and provision, but also to live in a relationship with the Holy Spirit. We must embrace the Holy Spirit as our helper, friend, and constant companion.

If you spend enough time in Christian circles, you will likely hear this battle referred to as walking in the flesh versus walking in the Spirit. I understand these may seem like peculiar, churchy terms, so let me explain.

Fundamental Christian Beliefs:

- When we accept Jesus as our Savior, the Holy Spirit comes to live within us (Ephesians 1:13-14).
- We now have access to the same power that raised Christ from the dead (Romans 8:11).
- We are free from the power of sin and death (Romans 8:2).
- We are no longer held captive by our sinful nature (Romans 7:6).

With all this in mind, we should follow the promptings and direction of the Holy Spirit living within us. Our sinful nature is at war with the Spirit. Galatians 5:17 NLT says, "...These two forces are constantly fighting each other, so you are not free to carry out your good intentions." The challenge is that many do not understand who the Holy Spirit is, much less how to walk in the Spirit.

The sad reality is that many believers live their lives never experiencing the blessings available from a relationship with the Holy Spirit. Far too often, believers experience the life-changing power of the Holy Spirit yet continue to live as if He does not exist. Upon believing in

Jesus, they acknowledge the Holy Spirit and experience His saving power at work within them, Ephesians 3:20-21 NIV. Yet, they continue to live on their own. A life lived by human strength for selfish motives is known as living in the flesh.

> "Far too often, believers experience the life-changing power of the Holy Spirit but go on living their lives as if He does not exist."
> Craig Booker

Listening To Your Body

Over the last several years, the reality of poor mental health has gone mainstream. Amid a global pandemic with new work and social protocols, poor mental health has become as common as unhealthy eating or sleeping habits. Fear and anxiety are showing up in the middle of church pews, and followers of Jesus are seeking ways to love others, including those with fear and anxiety, just as Jesus loved us. With the increasing complexities of life, people are now realizing the importance of mental health.

Warning! What I say in this chapter could offend many of my readers. Some things are hard to hear, let alone admit. I know this because I went through the same struggle of accepting this truth. I am not here to convince you that this applies to your situation; rather, I want to share my experience.

<u>Mental health is complex.</u>

A NEW PERSPECTIVE

Know that this certainly does not apply to all anxiety and fear. We should avoid using blanket statements about mental health. Each person's experience is unique and should be assessed on a case-by-case basis.

As believers, we are not designed for self-sufficiency. I have often found that fear and anxiety are signs. They serve as reminders, clues, and taps on the shoulder meant to show me that I am relying too much on myself. This is not a reason to feel embarrassed or ashamed. My body is signaling that I'm doing life wrong.

In the previous section of this chapter, I discussed the battle commonly referred to as living by the flesh versus walking in the Spirit. Every believer faces this challenge. Living according to our flesh often leaves us exhausted, frustrated, and empty. Furthermore, we miss out on an intimate relationship with God. When we neglect this relationship, we forfeit the abundant life that such a relationship with God offers.

Dependent By Design

Many believers believe that our choice to follow Jesus transforms us. We are different people, living our lives from a new source of truth, and holding a new worldview. We only have to look at 2 Corinthians 5:17 NLT to see that "...anyone who belongs to Christ has become a new person. The old life is gone; a new life has begun!" From this, we can safely say that following Jesus changes everything!

We should model our new life after God's perfect design. When God places a calling on our lives, He knows we cannot fulfill it on our own. This is by design. Our definition of success differs, and our approach to achieving it is also unique. We only need to look at John 15:4 to see that believers cannot be fruitful unless they remain in a relationship with Jesus, the vine (John 15:4-5).

God's calling on our lives requires the resources and fellowship of the Holy Spirit. Pursuing God's calling without the support and companionship of the Holy Spirit can lead to various downfalls, including exhaustion, frustration, and poor mental health.

A Recipe For Disaster

I am not suggesting that living in our strength leads to poor mental health. Much like our physical health, our mental health is influenced by various factors. These influences include, but are not limited to, genetics, biology, environment, trauma, and thoughts. I understand that brain health is not this simple, but I caution you against placing yourself in such a vulnerable position. Living out God's calling without the guidance of the Holy Spirit is a recipe for disaster.

In Acts 1:4-5, Jesus appears to his disciples during the 40 days following his resurrection. Before his ascension into heaven, he gave the disciples a command. The author of Acts highlights just one of the many things Jesus told them before ascending. Jesus commands the disciples, "Do not leave Jerusalem until the Father sends you the gift he promised..."

Think about this: During Jesus' time on earth, he gave his disciples one command as he prepared them for their ministry after his departure. One. One command stood out enough for the author of Acts to share it. This highlights the significance of the Holy Spirit in the lives of the disciples and in modern-day believers.

A NEW PERSPECTIVE

A Key Takeaway:
We should not live our lives apart from the Holy Spirit.

How Habits Impact Mental Health

Over the past 20 years, I have sought practical ways to improve my mental health. I am not against medication, but please do not suggest one that comes with a long list of side effects. Furthermore, I don't want to take an additional prescription to counteract the side effects of a new medication. And please, I beg you, please, do not tell me I don't have enough faith. All I want are some basic ways to improve my brain health.

While scientists and doctors may provide more detailed information on this topic, I have found the following to be beneficial. Quite frankly, this is the list I wish I had years ago. I fully believe in both medication and counseling and do not discount either. I want to be practical here. To be clear, I have not mastered all of these. I am learning to implement these strategies to improve my brain health.

Boundaries

Self-imposed boundaries can offer us freedom and a better way to live. Boundaries serve as healthy limits that prevent destructive behaviors in our lives and society. Establishing these guidelines requires both self-awareness and discipline. Successfully sticking to these limits is achieved through trial and error.

I admit, when I first started learning about the impact of diet, exercise, and sleep on my mental health, I was less than excited. In many ways, these areas are sources of comfort for me. Being told to instill boundaries felt like a complete loss. I am learning that embracing boundaries can lead to a fuller and more satisfying life.

Diet

The old cliché, "You are what you eat," seems truer now than ever. Every day, science reveals new insights into how food affects the human body. Admittedly, I don't like hearing that what I eat could negatively impact my health. Food often serves as a source of comfort, pleasure, and a safe space for me. Recognizing that the food I consume and when I eat may heighten anxiety is a critical piece of the puzzle.

It may sound strange, but I assure you that your body is trying to communicate with you. Whether or not you recognize it, your body provides clues about what is beneficial or detrimental to your health. After years of trial and error, I have tested these clues to see how small changes impact my health. Some of these experiments have led to breakthroughs, while others have not yielded any results.

Exercise

Most of us realize that exercise is beneficial. Whether we are trying to lose a few pounds or simply want to be in better shape, exercise is a fundamental way to improve our health. What if I told you that exercise also positively impacts mental health? Does this make implementing an exercise routine any easier? No, but it does offer a practical way to influence your mental health. It also helps improve the next area: sleep.

Sleep

I have struggled with maintaining good sleep hygiene for most of my life. By nature, I am a nighttime person. During my college years, this tendency was often beneficial for studying and enjoying downtime at the end of the day. However, after college, it proved to be more of a hindrance than anything.

A NEW PERSPECTIVE

While searching for treatment options for my mental health conditions, I was diagnosed with and began treatment for sleep apnea. After finding and adjusting to the treatment, I started to see how healthy sleep patterns positively impact my overall health. This process also revealed how damaging poor sleep hygiene can be when treating anxiety and depression. It became clear that if I wanted to get serious about addressing anxiety, I would need to confront my poor sleep habits.

The Choice Is Yours

Paying attention to your body's signals opens up practical options for enhancing your health. No one is forcing you to make these changes; the choice is yours. If you're anything like me, you seek practical ways to improve gradually. I would much rather heed my body's cues and safely experiment to discover what works than sit idly by and hope for the best.

Application Questions

1. In the chapter, I discuss the importance of identifying and processing trauma. How has addressing past traumas, or avoiding them, impacted your life or the lives of those around you? What challenges might one face when confronting their traumatic experiences?

2. The chapter emphasizes the tension between independence and reliance on the Holy Spirit for Christians. How do you balance self-reliance and dependence on God in your own life? Can you share an experience where you struggled with this balance?

3. In the chapter, I suggest that anxiety and fear can sometimes indicate that we're relying too heavily on ourselves rather than on God. Do you agree or disagree with this perspective? How might this view be helpful or potentially problematic when addressing mental health issues?

4. The chapter examines the impact of habits, including diet, exercise, and sleep, on mental health. Which of these areas do you find most challenging to manage, and why? Can you share any personal experiences in which changing one of these habits positively impacted your mental well-being?

4

Wellness, Well-being, & Why They Matter

Far too often, when we hear the word "health," our minds jump to physical health, such as exercise routines, diets, and disease prevention. Western culture, shaped by medical advancements and corporate wellness initiatives, has conditioned us to equate health with the absence of disease. But what if there's more to the picture? What if proper health—true well-being—involves more than just our physical bodies?

For Christians, this broader view of wellness is not only helpful; it is essential. We are not just physical beings—we are mind, body, and spirit, and God cares about our entire being.

A NEW PERSPECTIVE

What Is Wellness?

Wellness is the active pursuit of health. The National Wellness Institute defines it as "an active process through which people become aware of, and make choices toward, a more successful existence."[2] It includes the choices we make daily to nourish our bodies, minds, and spirits.

Unfortunately, wellness in our modern world is often reduced to corporate checklists: get your steps in, watch your weight, manage your stress, mainly for the sake of productivity. While these have value, they often overlook deeper dimensions of who we are. Historically, wellness has its roots in ancient practices such as Ayurveda and Traditional Chinese Medicine, both of which emphasize the harmony between the body, mind, and environment. In the same way, Scripture reminds us that caring for ourselves is not a new idea: "Do you not know that your bodies are temples of the Holy Spirit, who is in you..." (1 Corinthians 6:19 NIV).

What Is Well-being?

Well-being is a broader, more holistic concept. According to the World Health Organization, well-being is "a positive state experienced by individuals and societies."[3] It's not merely about preventing illness but about flourishing—experiencing purpose, peace, and resilience.

Think of well-being as a garden: it's not just about removing weeds (problems), but about cultivating growth, joy, connection, meaning, and rest.

It includes:

- **Physical Well-being:** Caring for our bodies through rest, movement, nutrition, energy levels, and sleep quality.

- **Mental & Emotional Well-being:** The ability to manage stress, cope with challenges, and maintain emotional stability, even during difficult times.

- **Spiritual Well-being:** Finding purpose and connection through faith, prayer, and living according to God's design.

- **Social Well-being:** Building meaningful relationships and participating in a supportive community of believers and friends.

- **Career & Financial Well-being:** Finding fulfillment in work and stewarding resources in ways that reduce stress rather than create it.

- **Environmental & Societal Well-being:** Living in harmony with our surroundings and contributing to God's kingdom on earth.

A person can exercise regularly, eat nutritious foods, and maintain healthy physical metrics, yet still struggle with loneliness, spiritual emptiness, or a lack of purpose, ultimately leading to poor overall well-being. This is especially relevant for those facing brain health challenges, where addressing only physical symptoms misses crucial elements of healing.

A NEW PERSPECTIVE

Why They Matter

When it comes to brain health challenges, there is no magic pill, simple solution, or quick fix. One size certainly does not fit all when it comes to treatment and recovery. A person struggling with their mental health wants—and needs—options. The first step toward recovery begins with understanding those options.

Wellness is an integral part of well-being, but it represents only one piece of the larger puzzle. Well-being is multi-dimensional, and what works for one person might not work for another. The more we learn about the factors that affect well-being, the better our chances of addressing the root causes of brain health challenges.

I recognize that this exploration of wellness and well-being has not been in-depth; it only scratches the surface. I am not a doctor, counselor, or psychologist, but I have done my best to summarize the material based on my research and personal experience. Some of this information was admittedly beyond my expertise, but I learned a great deal about what contributes to well-being, and I hope you have as well.

If there's one thing I want you to take away from this chapter, it's that you have choices in how you pursue well-being. There is no single right path, but rather a collection of strategies that can work together to create a healthier, more fulfilling life.

Faith, Well-being, & Brain Health

As someone who has navigated mental health challenges, I've learned that faith is central, not peripheral, to my well-being. While no single treatment or method guarantees healing, God's presence in our struggles offers peace and hope. The Bible reminds us that our bodies are temples (1 Corinthians 6:19-20), and caring for them includes nurturing our minds and spirits. Well-being is about alignment—our physical, mental, and spiritual selves working together in God's design.

Practical Steps for a Healthier Mind & Life

I've included some practical steps, grounded in a Christian perspective, that can help you move toward greater well-being, particularly in the context of brain health challenges:

1. **Prioritize Rest:** God Himself modeled the importance of rest (Genesis 2:2). Sleep, Sabbath observance, and time away from stressors are essential for physical and mental renewal.

2. **Move with Purpose:** Exercise isn't about performance—it's about well-being. Movement can enhance brain health, improve mood, and reduce stress.

3. **Feed Your Mind:** Scripture renews our thoughts (Romans 12:2). Engage with truth, seek godly wisdom, and pursue what is uplifting.

4. **Build Community:** Healing rarely happens in isolation. Reach out, connect, and let others carry the load with you (Galatians 6:2).

5. **Trust the Process:** Recovery takes time, patience, and grace. Be kind to yourself. God is not in a hurry, and He is faithful to complete the work He began in you (Philippians 1:6). As Paul reminds us in 2 Corinthians 12:9, God's power is made perfect in weakness.

Final Thoughts

Well-being is deeply personal, and what works for one person may not work for another. The more we understand what contributes to an abundant life, the better equipped we are to address brain health challenges with wisdom and faith.

If you're supporting someone facing brain health challenges, remember that your presence matters more than finding the perfect solution. Creating space for honest conversation, offering practical help without judgment, and patiently walking alongside someone through their journey can be a profound expression of Christ's love.

When we expand our understanding of health beyond mere wellness to embrace whole-person well-being, we open ourselves to God's comprehensive work in our lives. Even amidst ongoing struggles, we can experience growth, purpose, and moments of profound peace as we align our approach to health with God's design for human flourishing.

Application Questions

1. Reflecting on the chapter's discussion of wellness and well-being, how has your understanding of "health" evolved? In what ways do you see the concepts of wellness and well-being integrated—or not integrated—into your daily life?

2. The chapter emphasizes that wellness is only one facet of the broader concept of well-being. Consider the six dimensions of well-being (physical, mental/emotional, spiritual, social, career/financial, and environmental/societal). Which dimension do you believe is your strongest? Which dimension do you feel needs the most attention and why?

3. In what ways does your faith influence your approach to wellness and well-being? How might incorporating spiritual practices such as prayer, meditation, or worship contribute to your overall well-being?

A NEW PERSPECTIVE

4. The chapter outlines several practical steps for enhancing well-being, including prioritizing rest, purposeful movement, feeding your mind, building community, and trusting the process. Choose two of these steps and describe how you could implement them more effectively in your life. What challenges might you face, and how can you overcome them?

5. In the chapter, I share my perspective as someone who navigates mental health challenges, emphasizing the importance of faith and a holistic approach to well-being. If you or someone you know is facing similar challenges, what insights from this chapter resonate most? How might these insights inform your approach to seeking support and fostering healing?

6. The chapter highlights the significance of community in supporting individuals facing brain health challenges. How can you create or contribute to a supportive community within your sphere of influence (e.g., family, friends, church, workplace) to promote well-being and offer compassionate support to those in need?

5

Conversations for Good

As someone who has faced significant challenges with brain health, it can be daunting to think about how I could make an impact on our world. This book began with my desire to share my story in the hope of helping others who face similar challenges. It left me with many questions. While I understand this book may not change the world, I hope it marks the beginning of something much bigger than a book on your shelf.

Here are some of the questions I wrestled with:

- How could I shine a light in a dark world?

- What could I do to change a system that seems so broken?

- How do I help others who are facing these challenges?

- How can I support those who are helping others face these challenges?

In the following pages, I aim to contribute positively to the conversation about brain health. I want to initiate a dialogue that leads to progress for my community and others worldwide. I have developed a framework to shape our approach to discussing mental health with those around us. This framework is neither set in stone nor fixed. Additionally, I do not have it all figured out.

Consider this framework more as a first or second draft. It has substance but will require revision as we learn what works and what doesn't. I am always open to hearing your thoughts and input. If you would like to share your ideas, please contact me at craigbooker.com.

If you've made it this far in the book, thank you for investing your time and energy in better understanding mental health and its relationship to our world and faith in Jesus Christ. Whether you have experienced mental health challenges yourself or care about someone who has, you have taken a significant step toward improving the world around you. It may seem small, but it marks the beginning of something important.

Public Perception

Have you ever noticed that engaging in constructive conversations about mental health is challenging? Firstly, mental health is a broad topic that includes a wide range of issues. Can you imagine having a similar discussion about physical health? Secondly, everyone's experience with mental health is unique. While we can observe some similarities, making direct comparisons can be difficult.

The need for positive public conversations about mental health has never been more urgent. Adverse outcomes of poor mental health seem to seep from every crack and crevice in our society. In the United States, access to mental health care currently favors the wealthy. The societal stigma surrounding mental health remains incredibly strong despite significant progress.

Those responsible for creating policies and programs to serve our communities seem more interested in using current events to advance their political ambitions. Instead of serving the community, they prioritize their political party or personal interests. First-time politicians preach about serving "people like me," only to become just like the career politicians they ran against. Partisan politics hinder progress, pushing positive change into the future.

Uniting For Good

With all these challenges, how can we, as individuals, advocate for those we love? How do we discuss topics that divide us in pursuit of progress? Can we set aside our differences to achieve positive outcomes? Can we identify shared goals that transcend the political divide? If so, where do we begin? It's a complex question, but finding common ground is crucial.

Here are some strategies that might help:

- **Identify Shared Values:** Emphasize the values that individuals with differing political views share, such as the desire for healthy communities, thriving families, and a better future for the next generation. Present mental health as a universal concern that impacts all of these areas.

- **Emphasize the Economic Impact:** Poor mental health has significant economic consequences, including lost productivity, increased healthcare costs, and strain on social services. Presenting data and statistics on these costs can help depoliticize the issue and highlight the benefits of investing in mental health care.

- **Share Personal Stories:** Stories can be powerful tools for building empathy and understanding. Encourage individuals to share their own experiences with mental health challenges or the experiences of their loved ones. These narratives can help to humanize the issue and dismantle stereotypes.

- **Find Common Ground Initiatives:** Seek out or establish local initiatives that unite people across the political spectrum to support mental health. This could include community walks, awareness campaigns, or advocacy groups.

- **Start with dialogue:** Encourage respectful discussion in your community, whether at your church, local community center, or among your friends.

Everyday Conversations

We must begin with our conversation. By this, I mean the everyday interactions and activities that people engage in during their daily routines. Mental health is inextricably linked to our physical health. Mental health, including fear, anxiety, and depression, to name a few, is part of the larger conversation on health.

Mental Health = Brain Health

If you think about it, our brains are at the center of mental health. The human brain is part of our physical body. So why should we separate mental health from physical health? Instead, I prefer to call mental health by a different and more descriptive name. I believe the phrase "brain health" paints a more accurate picture.

The F.E.A.R. Framework

Seeking a more effective approach to discussing a healthy relationship with fear and anxiety, I developed the acronym F.E.A.R. At its core, the FEAR framework consists of four components, each of which has helped me cultivate a healthier relationship with fear.

Here's a more detailed look at the F.E.A.R. framework:

- **F - FOUNDATION:** Understanding your personal history with fear and anxiety, including past experiences, beliefs, and relationships. This also includes your relationship with God.

- **E - EDUCATION:** Learning about the nature of fear and anxiety, how they work, and their impact on your mind and body.

- **A - AWARENESS:** Developing a keen sense of your own thoughts, feelings, and behaviors related to fear and anxiety in the present moment. This includes self-awareness, awareness of the spiritual battle, and awareness of the "enemy."

- **R - RESOURCES:** Identifying and utilizing the support systems, tools, and practices that can help you cope with fear and anxiety.

I am not suggesting that knowing your past or being educated about fear solves all problems. Understanding your experiences with fear better prepares you to deal with what lies ahead. Gaining insight into past experiences and fear education paves the way for positive mental health. Armed with this knowledge, a person can make healthier choices.

A NEW PERSPECTIVE

Experience represents an individual's journey with fear and anxiety. Merging both our knowledge and awareness forms the basis of healthy living.

1. (F) FOUNDATION

An essential part of learning to cope with fear or anxiety in a healthy way begins with understanding our foundation. Our foundation encompasses personal experiences with fear and anxiety, as well as an individual's relationship with God. The foundation of any fear relationship consists of two components.

The Foundation:

- Fear Story - Our experience with fear
- Relationship with God

Fear Story

Everyone's experience with fear is unique. One of the first things we must realize is that everyone views life from their own perspective. This lens is often established in our youth and is regularly shaped by our thoughts, experiences, the people around us, and our environment. The same factors that shape our perspective also influence our fear story.

Understanding your fear story better prepares you for the road ahead. Many elements contribute to a fear story. We must examine the key events, people, and circumstances that shape our worldview. While we won't delve into the process of solidifying your fear story, we want to highlight three key areas that are essential to consider. Mapping out your trauma, triggers, and tendencies will significantly improve your mental health.

Fear Story: *A fear story encompasses the collective thoughts, experiences, events, circumstances, people, and environment that shape an individual's worldview.*

The 3 T's Of Your Fear Story

Understanding your fear story teaches you about past trauma, potential triggers, and behavioral tendencies. Being aware of past trauma, triggers, and tendencies better prepares you for the road ahead. Sharing these with a trusted friend or family member allows them to "have your back" when life gets tough.

3 T's Of Your Fear Story:

- **Trauma:** Events, circumstances, or people negatively impacting how you view the world.

- **Triggers:** Emotions or circumstances that can evoke fear and anxiety.

- **Tendencies:** Behaviors or thought patterns you lean towards given a set of circumstances.

Understanding your fear story will better equip you to face challenges on the road ahead. You may have encountered circumstances or traumas in your past that contribute to your anxiety. This process will help you recognize events, circumstances, and emotions that might trigger future anxiety. Knowing your fear story is a distinct advantage.

A NEW PERSPECTIVE

How does understanding my experience with fear and anxiety help?

Most people want to answer this question before investing time in understanding their past. Fear and anxiety are challenging enough the first time around. Why would anyone choose to revisit any of that? While I understand the feelings of resistance behind the question, I must reassure you that this is part of the process. To progress in the fight against fear and anxiety, we must gain a better understanding of our past.

Trauma & Triggers

I dive deep into the rest of my story in the chapter titled "What Got Me Here." Still, I hope this example proves helpful in illustrating this concept. In the past, I experienced trauma in finding a job that changed me forever. Anytime I look for a job, apply for a position, or go for an interview, I encounter extreme anxiety. I can shift from low anxiety to high alert in just a few minutes.

Finding a job stirs up the trauma I experienced during past job searches. The circumstances surrounding job searches trigger emotions from the fear and stress I encountered during a particular season. Understanding this aspect of my story prepares me for future job searches. It allows me to implement support measures if I foresee a job search on the horizon.

Tendencies

I hate to think of myself as predictable. In my younger years, being described as predictable would have been the equivalent of saying I am boring. As I have grown in age and wisdom, I realize that most humans exhibit certain behaviors or inclinations. Given a set of circumstances, many people tend to behave in a certain way.

tendency[4] [ten-duhn-see]

1. a natural or prevailing disposition to move, proceed, or act in some direction or toward

2. some point, end, or result: the tendency of falling bodies toward the earth.

3. an inclination, bent, or predisposition to something: a tendency to talk too much.

4. a special and definite purpose in a novel or other literary work.

As I have learned more about my mental health, I have noticed these tendencies emerging in my behavior. I do not always act in the same way, but there is typically a pattern to my actions. Understanding and maintaining awareness of my tendencies allows me to identify times when I might need help. It also enables me to enlist the support of friends and family members.

All this learning about tendencies is interesting, but it truly shines when enlisting the help of friends or family members. In your battle against fear or anxiety, you will need the support of those around you. Understanding and communicating your tendencies is a significant way for them to equip and protect you. They can more easily identify behavioral patterns or circumstances that might trigger anxiety.

How do I understand my fear & anxiety?

Gaining a better understanding of the fear and anxiety in your life does not have to be complicated. I will suggest a few options, but please understand there are others.

A NEW PERSPECTIVE

1. Find A Counselor

I recommend finding a trustworthy counselor to help you understand your fear story. This process was essential in aiding my understanding of my fear story. Remember that you are not committing to seeing this counselor indefinitely. You can choose to move on at any time.

2. Talk To Someone You Trust

There are times when a counselor is not accessible to everyone. A close, trusted friend or a church pastor can be equally beneficial.

3. Go Through A Book Or Study With A Group

While I have yet to learn of a specific study that focuses on discovering your fear story, one study I went through proved beneficial. The study was titled "Chazown" by Craig Groeschel. "Chazown" helps people find their God-given purpose. During this study, I uncovered milestone events that contributed to my purpose and the fears in my life. Tracing these events was vital to understanding how my past influences my future.

Combining Methods

I took what I learned through Chazown to my counselor, and we discussed it in greater detail. These sessions helped me process the milestones that play a pivotal role in my life today. The practice of mapping out life events provided me with a visual timeline that I still refer to today.

Understand that this process never ends. Reviewing the results has greatly helped me understand what I found, but I still find myself returning to specific areas of my story. These exercises serve as a starting point, a foundation for comprehending my journey. Please do your best, but don't feel pressured to complete it in one attempt. Inevitably, you will uncover details later that you overlooked in previous sessions. It is essential to keep this information close at hand so that you can revisit it.

Your Relationship With God

I need to explain how much I resisted discussing faith as part of the foundation of the fear framework. I wanted to include everyone. If I leave out faith in Christ as part of the framework, I might welcome more people, but I would be deceiving my core audience. One lesson I have learned in writing this book is to know your audience and speak directly to that audience. This is the key to successfully serving them.

Here is what I can tell you. I tried to fight fear without God. I truly tried. Not because I am noble or brave or seek a challenge, but out of fear! I was afraid that if I depended on Jesus and the attempt failed, I would lose my faith. It sounds silly, but I could not risk it. I needed my faith; no matter how ridiculous it seemed, I would do anything to protect it. The truth is, I was undermining my faith, not protecting it.

Stop Here

I understand if this turns you off or if you decide to stop reading this book here. I get it. I won't blame you for putting this down because I brought Jesus Christ into the picture. If you prefer to search for another book that promises freedom from fear and anxiety without Jesus, please feel free to move on.

A NEW PERSPECTIVE

The reality of life without Jesus should fill you with fear. We try to convince ourselves that we can live this life without God's help. You could even go so far as to say that there are many ways to heaven. Numerous books in the world argue both sides of this position. Check them out and determine what you believe.

I created this book with a relationship with Jesus Christ as the main ingredient. So, if this is your stop, I respect that. I would prefer you stop rather than get to the end and think, "Is that all he's got?" I wish you nothing but the best.

If you still choose to interact with me through my website, email, and social media, I will do everything I can to help you. My assistance is not conditional on your faith in Jesus Christ. Love remains my motivator. I will do all I can, out of love, to support you along the way.

Promises, Promises

Many more promising options are available to you by placing your faith in Christ. I just won't pretend that it makes everything better. Choosing to follow Jesus does not offer freedom from trials, but it comes with many invaluable promises from God. The Holy Spirit will come to live inside you—the same Spirit who raised Jesus Christ from the dead. Jesus will always be with you, so you never face this world alone. I can tell you there will be unexplainable peace and joy in many of your trials. God will answer prayers you did not know to pray. Sometimes, you wonder if God is still there until something happens that only God can explain.

Batteries Not Included

Did you ever receive a fantastic gift, only to find out that the person who gave it to you forgot to include the batteries? You open the instructions to discover that the gift requires one of those strange, uncommon batteries, the kind only found at a specialty battery store. This isn't as much of an issue today with one-day delivery and stores being open on or around the holidays.

Back when I was a kid, we sometimes had to wait one or more days before we could purchase the much-needed batteries. The wait felt like torture! I could see the gift, touch it, and even mimic what it did, but it wasn't the same without the batteries.
The gift was incomplete.

The advice, tips, and insights I have to share on fear and anxiety are valuable, but they are not the same without a relationship with Jesus. The suggestions that do not involve faith play a small part in a rich and satisfying life.

> **Warning:** *Without a relationship with Jesus, they may be lacking, much like a gift without batteries. At the core of your struggle with fear lies a spiritual component that can only be satisfied through a relationship with Jesus Christ.*

2. (E) EDUCATION

Learning about fear, anxiety, and mental illness is one of the most powerful tools for pursuing better mental health. As a kid and even as an adult, I have always longed to understand how things work. I used to take things apart to learn their mechanics. I would then reassemble the item and test it again to ensure that I had not broken anything. Understanding the inner workings of electronics, tools, and computer programs has provided me with a certain satisfaction.

Once you have a basic understanding of how an item works, you can troubleshoot problems more effectively. Although the inner workings of the human brain are far

A NEW PERSPECTIVE

more complex than those of a tool or electronic device, the concept still applies. Having basic knowledge of fear, anxiety, and mental health can significantly aid in resolving issues. This concept should empower you, but it does not replace the need to seek help. Education is a tool.

The Role Of Education

My goal for this section is not to educate readers on all the science behind fear and anxiety. Doctors and counselors are better suited to take on that task. I hope to highlight the importance of education in your pursuit of better mental health. Don't overlook this piece of the puzzle.

Here are some key areas to focus on in your education:

- **The Biology of Fear and Anxiety:** Understanding the brain structures and neurochemicals involved in the fear response can help you realize that these feelings are not merely a matter of willpower.

- **Common Mental Health Conditions:** Learning about conditions such as generalized anxiety disorder, panic disorder, social anxiety disorder, and depression can help you recognize symptoms in yourself or others and seek appropriate help.

- **Coping Mechanisms:** Researching healthy coping strategies, such as mindfulness, deep breathing exercises, and progressive muscle relaxation, can offer you practical tools for managing anxiety in the moment.

- **The Impact of Trauma:** If your fear and anxiety stem from past trauma, learning about the effects of trauma on the brain and body can be a crucial step in your healing process.

- **The Mental Health System:** Understanding how to navigate the mental health care system, including different types of providers, treatment options, and insurance coverage, can empower you to make informed decisions about your care.

3. (A) AWARENESS

Living with awareness is key to maintaining a healthy relationship with fear and anxiety. A significant part of this involves self-awareness, but it doesn't stop there. While it is essential to understand our Fear Story, it also involves an awareness of the spiritual battle. Awareness marks the beginning of the battle, so let's get started.

Areas of Awareness:

- Your Fear Story
- Fear & Anxiety - The Spiritual Battle
- The Enemy

Your Fear Story

Understanding your Fear Story is crucial for confronting anxiety. For many years, I went through life without this knowledge. I was unaware of my trauma, triggers, or patterns that led me down this path. I found myself reacting to circumstances, stress, fear, and anxiety.
I often felt overwhelmed, fatigued, and lacking resources to navigate life.

A NEW PERSPECTIVE

An awareness of your Fear Story results from significant effort. One invests considerable time in uncovering trauma, triggers, and tendencies to reach this point. The process often involves revisiting complex past events and unearthing old wounds you may have buried long ago. Understand that the time and energy spent here can yield exponential rewards.

Fear Story - The 3 T's:

- Trauma
- Triggers
- Tendencies

Understanding trauma, triggers, and tendencies will not magically resolve issues, but it enables individuals to prepare. Similar to preparing for a major exam, one often reviews a study guide or enrolls in a test prep course to perform at their best. Soldiers heading into battle will study the terrain and their adversaries to devise a strategic plan. Preparation does not guarantee success, but it significantly enhances your chances.

Fear & Anxiety - The Spiritual Battle

I understand what it's like to live with a healthy balance of fear and anxiety. My relationship with fear has been positive for over half of my life. Fear has properly informed my decisions for a long time but has not ruled my life. So why do I struggle to restore balance and make choices that reflect my true beliefs? Why do I grapple so much with ordinary decisions?

Everyone has a somewhat unique relationship with fear. Once fear took hold of me, dealing with it became completely different. I remember a time when fear might have influenced my decisions, but not as much as it does now. I see that sometimes dread, looming disaster, or failure are just emotions. At other times, a clear battle is brewing.

The Spiritual Battle

There are two parts to the spiritual battle of fear and anxiety.

1. Facing Fear In The Moment - Short Term

2. A Look At The Big Picture Battle - Long Term

1. Facing Fear In The Moment

Awareness:

How To Prepare For Spiritual Battle

Part of the battle is recognizing that some days, overwhelming feelings are just that - feelings. They are valid and deserving of your time and attention. However, not every struggle with fear stems from the Enemy's attacks. Conversely, there will be days when the situation involves more than just feelings or emotions. So, what do we do?

I want to avoid over-dramatizing fear scenarios by suggesting that every occurrence comes from the Enemy. Determining whether a spiritual battle is at play is a learning process that lies outside the scope of this

A NEW PERSPECTIVE

book. Instead of focusing on the Enemy, I prefer to provide you with a practical strategy you can implement today.

I encourage you to approach every occurrence in a similar way, and I'll explain why. Dealing with fear in the heat of the moment is challenging enough. Having one clear strategy will simplify your response.

Fear Strategy

- Take the situation to God in prayer.

- Phone a friend (via text or phone)

Take It From Me To We

Fear grows best in isolation. When we take the struggle from me to we, a shift occurs. Bringing the situation to God in prayer places the fight and the outcome in God's hands. Calling a friend is like recruiting soldiers for battle. Both actions are essential, but the first is a game-changer.

Amid the mess, we are making a statement of faith. This action conveys our trust in God and acknowledges that this situation is bigger than ourselves. We place our trust in Him regarding the situation and its outcomes. Not only does this please God, but it also alleviates the pressure on us.

I get it. The last thing you want to do is be vulnerable by sharing your fear with others. The fear is difficult enough as it stands. Trust me; I wouldn't ask you to be vulnerable if there were a better option.

Weaken Fear's Foundation By Removing Isolation

After presenting your fear to God in prayer, embracing vulnerability is the most powerful action you can take. When we invite a friend into our fear, several things happen.

Steps To Remove Isolation

- We shine a light on fear by telling a friend.
- We harness the power of community.

Fear always makes the most sense when we keep it to ourselves. When we share our fear with a friend, we open ourselves to recognizing its flaws. A friend can help us see things from a fresh perspective. Lies become apparent when we bring them into the open. A friend can help us see the lies we are believing objectively.

Being part of a community doesn't mean you have to share your fears with strangers. It means you don't have to face your fears alone. Whether you confide in one friend or several, opening up allows God to work through others. Your community can offer encouragement, support, and help during your recovery.

Be sure to identify a friend or multiple friends you can reach out to in advance. Talk with them to communicate what you need in these moments. Setting expectations with them will prepare them to support you when you need it. It would not be ethical to suggest I have mastered this process.

A NEW PERSPECTIVE

I still need help with it, but I'm sharing what I've learned so far. In part 1, "Facing Fear In The Moment," I encouraged you to approach every fear scenario similarly. My goal is to offer practical applications rather than discuss theory or nuances. This will give you a tangible strategy to face your fears.

2. The Larger Battle

Now, we will focus more on the less tangible things I have learned. Here, I'll draw upon my personal experience and the Biblical concept of walking in the flesh versus the spirit. The longer I engage with this, the more I notice the spiritual battle between my human desires (the flesh) and following the Spirit. It's challenging to address this topic effectively on multiple levels within the context of this book, so I am sharing only from my experience.

Whenever we face fear, we can choose to put our faith in God or human desires. Christians refer to this as walking in the Spirit versus the flesh. This battle involves choosing between following human emotions, desires, and inclinations or those that align with God's will. Here, I will discuss how the struggle between the flesh and the Spirit uniquely impacts those dealing with fear and anxiety.

Believers who struggle with overwhelming fear and anxiety due to trauma, circumstances, or experiences uniquely encounter this flesh versus Spirit battle. As they strive to reclaim a sense of safety, they often isolate themselves from the world. They tend to react to situations or requests by seeking safety and protection, shielding themselves from potential harm. This need for security can quickly overshadow other priorities.

As followers of Jesus, the Bible teaches Christians to love God and others above themselves. In your walk, God will often lead you to situations that require action. The decision to obey God's promptings becomes increasingly challenging when safety is the number one priority. Christians who deal with anxiety must choose between their hyperactive need for security and obedience, as well as the fundamentals of their faith.

Anyone who has experienced trauma or challenging circumstances resulting in anxiety may need to take steps to restore their sense of safety. Scaling back activities and responsibilities can be helpful as they practice self-care. Eventually, they must begin taking small steps back into the real world. This practice is vital to help them get out of their heads and prevent new areas of fear from emerging.

What was once a good, healthy idea can become a significant obstacle in a person's life. If left unchecked, the need for perceived safety can supersede everything else, robbing the individual of any chance for a rich and satisfying life. The more this person shields themselves from the world, the greater the likelihood of their fears growing or appearing in new areas. They must take gradual, small steps to change their way of thinking.

The Push For Control & Certainty

After experiencing trauma or loss, it is common to feel overwhelming fear and anxiety. Our human desires (the flesh) desperately seek control and certainty—the greater the level of fear and anxiety, the more our flesh craves these two things.

A NEW PERSPECTIVE

The more we struggle to feel safe, the more we limit our exposure to outside influences. Inadvertently, we forfeit the opportunity for a rich, fulfilling life in pursuit of an existence devoid of risk. The longer we attempt to control, the clearer it becomes that we cannot control everything. We are trying to create a reality that doesn't exist.

Let me paint a picture of how this false reality might appear. Yours may differ according to your Fear Story, but the concept remains the same. As you can see, the requirements are unrealistic and absurd. Living life to avoid fear and anxiety is not truly living at all.

Our False Reality (An Example):

Career:

- Self-sufficient
- Be self-employed
- Work remotely

Romantic Relationships:

- It's all about you. The other person serves your interests
- They do not push back to meet their needs.

Friendships:

- You always get your way. They consistently strive to meet your needs for companionship.

Health:

- Be perfectly healthy, always.

Finances:

- Be independently wealthy
- We store up wealth for ourselves.
- We give when it is convenient.

Faith:

- God serves us; we don't serve him.

How Do We Explain These Desires?

After experiencing significant trauma or loss, we strive to make the world stop spinning. Like a rug, our sense of safety is pulled out from under our feet. We see danger everywhere we look. We long for the good old days when our world felt safer.

If we continue to face circumstances that threaten our sense of safety, we will desperately reach for more control. We begin to experience anxiety in new ways. We no longer enjoy the things we cherished only days or weeks ago. Going out to eat, going into the office, or visiting our favorite travel destination feels unreal.

As believers, our lack of safety makes trusting in God incredibly difficult. We feel conflicted about what we believe. We can experience significant shame as we struggle to embrace biblical truth. We may know certain

A NEW PERSPECTIVE

things in our minds, but putting them into practice becomes unthinkable. Our newfound feelings force us to choose between our emotions and our beliefs.

> "For the flesh desires what is contrary to the Spirit, and the Spirit what is contrary to the flesh. They are in conflict with each other, so that you are not to do whatever you want."
> Galatians 5:17 NIV

A Walking Contradiction

A life of control and certainty contradicts the life God calls believers to live. Not only does this go against God's plan for our lives, but it is also unrealistic. Regardless of a person's belief in God, attempting to control every aspect of our lives proves foolish. For believers, this path is contrary to following Jesus. One can pursue one or the other, but one cannot seek both.

I encourage you not to take my word for it; let us examine what the Bible says about how Christians live their lives. We will begin in Matthew 22, where a Pharisee, an expert in religious law, tries to trap Jesus with a question.

> "'Teacher, which is the most important commandment in the law of Moses?' Jesus replied, 'You must love the Lord your God with all your heart, all your soul, and all your mind.' This is the first and greatest commandment. A second is equally important: 'Love your neighbor as yourself.'"
> Matthew 22:36-39 NLT

God Calls All Believers
To Love God And Others

The most fundamental part of living out faith in Jesus Christ requires Christians to relinquish any possibility of control and certainty. Loving God with all your heart, soul, and mind means denying personal desires. Even if we ignore Jesus' command to love others, we cannot expect a life free of risk. Following Christ involves risking everything to love God with all our beings; likewise, loving your neighbor as yourself may require even greater risk.

The longer I live with this battle for control and certainty, the more apparent it becomes that living this way goes against what God has for my life. To obsess over control and certainty is to enslave oneself in a foolish pursuit and rob oneself of joy. While I deeply understand the trauma and emotions behind this desire, I have seen how this pursuit is a trap. It is a prison that only you can choose to escape.

> "It is for freedom that Christ has set us free. Stand firm, then, and do not let yourselves be burdened again by a yoke of slavery."
> Galatians 5:1 NIV

Please understand my words. I am not oversimplifying the process of walking out of this self-made prison. I face the decision to leave this way of thinking behind every day. Some days are easier than others, while on many days, I must claw my way out of this pit. I am intimately familiar with the struggle.

After witnessing how the pursuit of control and certainty robs me of joy, I pre-decided to choose a rich life over a "safe" one. I often ask questions like, "What am I giving up in this situation to feel safe?" "Will I look back on this situation and regret choosing the safe option?"

Specific questions like these help my brain shift from a fear mindset to an observer mindset. This process is still new to me, so I am not ready to discuss it at length.

The Enemy

Living with an awareness of the Enemy can be challenging. First, if the concept of a spiritual adversary is new to you, it is easy to develop a fascination with the Devil. Suddenly, you notice evidence of his work in many different areas of your life. Before you know it, you see his fingerprints everywhere you look.

This experience is much like buying a car. When purchasing a new vehicle, one might begin researching, looking at photos, and reading reviews. Suddenly, that person sees that model of car everywhere they turn. Those vehicles were always there, but their attention is now hyper-focused on them.

Resist Preoccupation

While learning to look out for our enemy is not a bad thing, I caution you not to become consumed by it. This fascination can easily distract you from living a life of purpose. It can also become a scapegoat for all the negative aspects of your life. Yes, the Enemy is actively working in our world, but he is not the cause of every adverse event in our lives.

> "Stay alert! Watch out for your great enemy, the devil. He prowls around like a roaring lion, looking for someone to devour. Stand firm against him, and be strong in your faith. Remember that your family of believers all over the world is going through the same kind of suffering you are."
> 1 Peter 5:8-9 NLT

To maintain a balanced perspective on the Enemy, consider these points:

- **Focus on God's Sovereignty:** Remember that God is ultimately in control, and the Enemy's power is limited.

- **Discernment, Not Delusion:** Develop discernment to recognize the Enemy's influence without attributing every difficulty to him.

- **Live a Purpose-Driven Life:** Keep your attention on your God-given purpose and calling, rather than fixating on the Enemy.

- **Community and Support:** Stay connected with your faith community for encouragement and accountability.

- **Spiritual Warfare is Real:** Acknowledge the reality of spiritual warfare, but don't let it consume your thoughts or dictate your actions.

4. (R) RESOURCES

I'll admit that reading about resources is not the most exciting activity. Still, this topic is more important than you might imagine. There are moments in my Fear Story when I desperately needed the right resources to help me cope with the circumstances I faced. There was so much about anxiety that I did not understand, and I also did not know where to turn in those moments.

A Variety Of Resources

Resource needs will vary depending on where you are in your journey. I will start by addressing those who are new to anxiety, but resources are essential at all stages. I prioritize helping those who are new to anxiety because I felt lost when I began down this path. I have created a section on my website to provide helpful resources. You can access it by visiting the resources section of my website craigbooker.com.

Out Of Reach

It can be challenging to think beyond your emotions when experiencing overwhelming anxiety for the first time. Knowing who to turn to or where to seek help often feels out of reach. In many cases, your family or friends may scramble to find the resources you need. They may feel overwhelmed in obtaining the necessary help unless they are familiar with the situation.

If your friends or family are fortunate enough to know someone who can guide you in the right direction, remember you are the exception. Most people will reach out to friends, family, and acquaintances in search of recommendations. At this stage, desperation for help often precedes finding the best resource for the individual in need. Should you contact a counselor or a physician, or both?

If you have a primary care physician, this is often a good place to begin. The doctor may not have all the answers, but they will probably be able to suggest options that can help. They will also perform a basic exam to get a thorough understanding of the patient's condition. This visit is likely the first of many on the path to finding help.

Visiting your doctor is not necessarily more important than finding a counselor. However, you'll probably be able to see them sooner. Unfortunately, getting help often takes longer than it should. Sadly, in most cases, insurance tends to cover a doctor's visit rather than counseling. I wish I had started the search for a counselor immediately after scheduling my doctor's appointment.

Group Therapy

For many, some form of group therapy can be helpful. Personally, hearing about others' mental health struggles was an eye-opener. Although it was enlightening, it also increased my anxiety and pushed me to a place I wasn't ready to explore. Maybe it was the wrong timing or setting, so I decided to skip this option for now. Having some form of accountability might be useful, but I haven't looked into it deeply yet. While I hope this framework helps others understand and talk about mental health, there's still a lot of work to do. For more resources, I suggest visiting craigbooker.com.

Application Questions

1. In the chapter, I discuss the concept of a "Fear Story" composed of trauma, triggers, and tendencies. How might understanding your own Fear Story help you better cope with anxiety and fear? Can you identify any key elements of your personal Fear Story?

2. The chapter emphasizes the importance of education in dealing with fear and anxiety. Why do you think learning about these topics is valuable? What are some ways you could educate yourself further about mental health?

3. In the chapter, I describe a spiritual battle between following human desires ("the flesh") versus God's will ("the Spirit") when dealing with fear. How do you view the relationship between faith and mental health struggles? Do you see any conflicts between seeking safety/control and living out your beliefs?

4. What are your thoughts on my suggestion to "take it from me to we" when facing fear - specifically by praying and reaching out to a friend? What potential benefits or challenges do you see in this approach?

5. How can public conversations about mental health be improved to reduce stigma and increase access to care?

6. How does personal experience shape one's understanding and management of fear and anxiety?

7. In what ways can individuals or communities advocate for mental health support despite political and societal challenges?

8. How does understanding your own 'Fear Story' help in managing anxiety, and how can this concept be applied in everyday life?

9. Reflecting on the F.E.A.R. framework, which component (Foundation, Education, Awareness, Resources) do you find most challenging to address in your own life, and why?

10. How can you apply the principles of the F.E.A.R. framework in your daily life to cultivate a healthier relationship with fear and anxiety?

Conclusion

Wow! You did it! Congratulations on sticking with it and reaching the end! Even though this book was pretty short, staying curious and open to learning more about brain health is a tough challenge. I also understand that if you or someone you know is facing brain health issues, your schedule and life can be very busy. It really means a lot that you took a little extra time in your day or week to improve your perspective.

When I started this book, I simply wanted to share my story in a way that gives others hope—hope that no matter what they are going through, healing is not only possible but also accessible. The challenge is that healing looks different for me than it does for everyone else. For me, the path toward healing will probably be quite different than it would be for you or someone you love.

CONCLUSION

Takeaways

In the quest to add value to your life and those around you, I ask myself questions like, "What bits of wisdom or encouragement could I offer?" What could I do to prepare you for the road ahead? If I could speak to myself back in the year 2000, what would I say? It's tough to fully prepare the younger me for what I would face over the following twenty-five-plus years. Here are a few of the big takeaways:

Do Not Give Up Hope

A common model for authors is to share their stories and show how others can apply what worked for them, but this would be a mistake. This approach often works brilliantly for certain topics, but not so for mental health. What works for one person often won't work for another. We can sometimes take bits and pieces from someone else's experience. Still, applying their entire approach to our unique challenges is tough. Instead of selling you on a formula, I beg you not to give up hope for recovery.

When it comes to trauma, anxiety, and depression, it's not like comparing apples to apples. Our uniqueness and our unique life experiences often make applying a single method of treatment a challenge. On top of that, I found that one treatment doesn't resolve every issue. I may make progress in one area and then wait months or even years to find progress in other areas.

I hope that you continue being open to new treatment options until you find something that works for you. This process can and will take weeks, months, or even years. I pray you will remain hopeful and curious to discover that recovery is possible if we don't give up. I also pray that you find a community to love and support you through this challenging process.

CONCLUSION

Resist

Resist the urge to compare your challenges with a neighbor, friend, or family member. Instead, be inspired by their story. Learn what you can from their battle, but don't be discouraged when what works for them doesn't work for you. Cheer for them and be grateful for the victory they have found. Their healing is proof that recovery is possible for you, too.

Avoid Assumptions

A common mistake many people make, including myself, is assuming what recovery and healing look like—assuming that healing for brain health challenges follows the same pattern as the common cold or the flu. Falsely believing that all we need to do is take some medicine and the illness will be gone in a week or two. I learned there is danger in making these types of assumptions.

In the past, I often believed I could return to how things used to be before all this happened. I thought that if I had faith, took my medication, and attended counseling, I could somehow miraculously go back to a time when brain health struggles weren't an issue. The problem is that I didn't realize how much I had changed. I assumed I could go back to being the person I once was, but that person no longer exists.

Try New Things

I encourage you to become a student of your body. Under the supervision of a doctor or counselor, be willing to try new things to find what works best for you. The process of experimenting, staying positive, and remaining curious as you search for methods to address your struggles is essential. It's more about a mindset than following a series of steps.

CONCLUSION

Find A Community

Out of all of the lessons I have learned along the way, one of the most important that will stick with me is the importance of community. For so long, I tried to go on this journey by myself. This was one of the most difficult things to learn.

We need people.

As an introvert who values time alone, I found this tough. Over the last few years, one of the best things I have done is to intentionally develop a community around me. I would love to say that this was entirely my idea, but it wasn't. I felt God's prompting to begin a community. He left me little signs or clues, but eventually, He held up a flashing neon sign that got my attention.

When I could no longer deny that God was behind these signs, I did it. I followed God's prompting to create Overflow. Overflow is a loving community where everyone understands the challenges associated with fear, anxiety, and depression. If you would like to learn more about Overflow, go to overflow.community.

So what?!?

Anytime I write something, whether it's an article, a newsletter, a script for a podcast, or a video for YouTube, I try to ask, "So what?" What difference does any of this make? Why should anyone care about this? What value did I add to the conversation? What is one thing that I

CONCLUSION

could do to make an impact on someone reading this book? I believe the biggest contribution I can make involves perspective.

A New Perspective

In the introduction of this book, I said what most people need before they visit a doctor or a counselor is a change in perspective. (I was exaggerating a little to make a point. I don't want you or someone else to avoid seeing a doctor, but I hope you understand the importance of perspective.) My journey with brain health has taught me that I always need to work on my perspective. This is not only applicable to brain health, but to your faith, and life itself. It's one of those lessons that I learn and need to keep learning as I go.

Look, I understand that you probably started reading or listening to this book in hopes of finding a secret formula, some shortcuts, or a map to help you through the mess of mental health. And while I would love to be able to provide those to you, it would be misleading at best. Any map I provided you would need to be custom-tailored to all the variables that make you, you. The process would be highly involved, and I would need supernatural help.

God is actively teaching you and me through all of the highs and lows. We learn how to connect with God and depend on him in ways we never thought possible. He teaches us the dangers of comparison and assumptions. We discover the importance of building Godly relationships around us. We learn how God is working to make all things new, including you and me. Hopefully, with all of these lessons, we see things in a slightly different light.

CONCLUSION

This is what we must hold onto. In this new perspective, we begin to see how God might use this collective experience to help others. He'll use wisdom from the messiest of moments to bless others who are hurting. In serving others, God will often do more than we could ask, think, or imagine.

So, here I leave you with a new perspective. I pray you will dig into this perspective and seek God for what He might teach you. I pray that you know you are not alone. I pray you know that this is only the beginning. While I have touched on many things, the conversation is far from over.

Acknowledgments

I want to express my gratitude and thank all my friends and family who made this book possible.

To Kristi Booker: what can I say? You've been my biggest fan as I chased my dream of becoming an author. The journey has been long, and you've stood by my side, cheering me on every step of the way! You have played every possible role in my quest to be an author. I love you more each day!

Kenley Booker: I finally did it! Thank you for always supporting me in my journey to become an author. You've listened to my endless stories about writing without ever seeming bored. So, bravo, and thank you!

Mom and Dad: thank you for supporting me, even when my wild ideas didn't make sense. Thank you for listening to me ramble about writing. Here's to an idea that finally worked out!

Jimmy and Debbie Pope: thank you for all your love and support. You have smiled and nodded, even when you were probably tired of hearing me talk about my writing journey.

ACKNOWLEDGMENTS

Margie Menlove: I can't express how much your friendship means to me. You've become one of my greatest supporters, and I thank God for having you in my life.

Nathan Yack: thank you for inviting me to serve in IT at Life.Church. Your one invitation has brought countless blessings into my life. Your ability to recognize something in me and invite me to serve has transformed my life.

Noel Lundy: who knew that serving together in IT at Life.Church would bring so many blessings? You're an incredible friend, and I truly appreciate your support.

Kurt Theyel: thank you for always being there to provide a voice of reason, offer wisdom, or listen when I need it most. You are such a great friend!

Tyler Wilkerson: it's fascinating how God brings the right people into our lives. While we served together, you recognized something in me that I didn't see, and I can't thank you enough for believing in me.

Sean McHargue: your friendship and confidence in me played such a crucial role in my recovery. You always believed in me and helped me in such a challenging season of my life.

Chris Morris: I can't believe I finally made it here! You've been an amazing friend and an invaluable source of encouragement on my journey to becoming an author.

Dustin Walker: you are an essential part of my support system. I can't imagine being well enough to write this book without you. Thank you for listening patiently and providing guidance when I need it.

ACKNOWLEDGMENTS

Craig Groeschel: you do not know me, but you have been my pastor and mentor for twenty-five years. You help me grow closer to God every week, and I would not be the same without your leadership, teaching, and encouragement. I am truly grateful to you and Amy for being such a godly example and leading with such generosity. Countless lives are different because of you!

Robyn Morrow: thank you for believing in me and supporting my writing even before anyone recognized me as a writer. You have always been there to support me, and I am truly grateful.

The Overflow Community: wow! This day has finally arrived. You've been incredibly supportive throughout my journey to becoming an author. Thank you for believing in me. Thank you for making the Overflow Community what it is today.

To you, the reader: thank you for taking a chance on me, and more importantly, for investing in your well-being and that of those around you.

Notes

Chapter 3: Milestones, Waypoints, & Life Lessons

1. Trauma Definition 1. The American Heritage® Dictionary of the English Language, 5th Edition.

Chapter 4: Wellness, Well-Being, & Why They Matter

2. National Wellness Institute. (n.d.). What is wellness? Retrieved from https://nationalwellness.org/resources/what-is-wellness/

3. World Health Organization. (n.d.). Well-being. Retrieved from https://www.who.int/news-room/fact-sheets/detail/mental-health-strengthening-our-response

Chapter 5: Conversations for Good

4. (n.d.). Tendency Definition. Dictionary.com. https://www.dictionary.com/browse/tendency

About the Author

Craig Booker is the founder of Overflow, a community that supports individuals dealing with anxiety, depression, and brain health challenges and their loved ones. He also serves as the Executive Director of Serve First Ministries, a nonprofit dedicated to helping people experience the radical blessings of serving others. As a writer and brain health advocate, Craig Booker is passionate about creating safe spaces that foster authenticity, love, growth, acceptance, and encouragement.

CB

Find additional resources on brain health, faith, and personal growth.

craigbooker.com

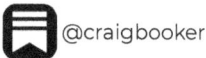 @craigbooker 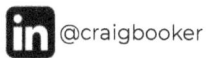 @craigbooker 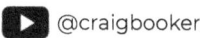 @craigbooker

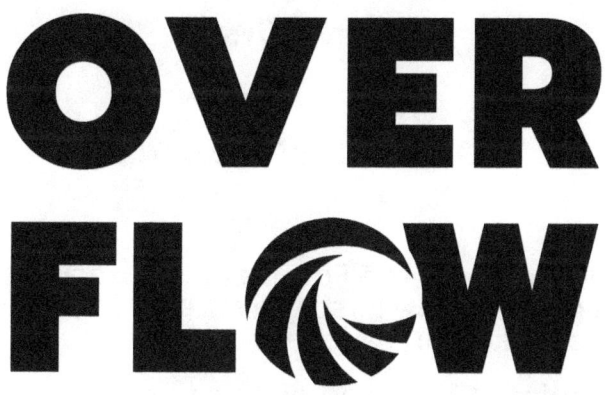

WITH CRIAG BOOKER

Subscribe to the **Overflow with Craig Booker Podcast** on Apple Podcasts or wherever you listen to podcasts.

Visit **www.overflow.community/podcast** to find episodes, videos, resources, and more.

 Apple Podcasts   Spotify

 Google Podcasts   YouTube

About Serve First

Craig Booker is the Founder and Executive Director of Serve First Ministries, a 501(c)(3) nonprofit organization.

Our mission is to lead people to experience the radical blessings of serving.

We achieve this through creative media, resources, and relationships.

If you were inspired by A New Perspective: A Journey of Brain Health, Faith, and Well-being, then you should explore what Serve First offers.

iservefirst.org

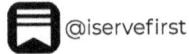 @iservefirst   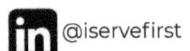 @iservefirst   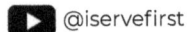 @iservefirst

OVER FLOW

OVERFLOW.COMMUNITY

Join a growing community learning about brain health, and following Jesus.

@overflowcommunity   @overflowcommunity

www.ingramcontent.com/pod-product-compliance
Lightning Source LLC
Chambersburg PA
CBHW020551030426
42337CB00013B/1045